HAIR RESTORATION PROCEDURES FOR BEGINNERS

Comprehensive Guide To Understanding, Choosing, And Mastering Effective Restoration Techniques, Treatments, And Solutions

DR SAWYER DIEGO

DISCLAMER

Nothing in this book should be interpreted as medical advice; it is meant exclusively for educational reasons. Regarding their specific health issues and treatment options, readers are urged to speak with licensed healthcare professionals. The publisher and author disclaim all liability for any errors or omissions in the material provided, as well as for any negative effects that may arise from using or abusing the information. Although every attempt has been taken to guarantee that the material in this book is correct as of the date of publishing, new research may have superseded some of the content because medical knowledge is always changing. It is recommended that readers confirm the most recent medical recommendations and guidelines. The reader of this book undertakes to release the author and publisher from any claims or liabilities resulting from the use of this information, and understands and accepts the inherent risks connected with healthcare decisions.

TABLE OF CONTENTS

ABOUT THE BOOK

"Hair Restoration Procedures for Beginners" is a thorough guide that offers readers a clear understanding of the complex reasons behind this common concern. By addressing the psychological impact of hair loss early on, the book sets a compassionate tone and acknowledges the emotional journey that often accompanies this experience. Understanding the profound impact of hair loss goes beyond mere aesthetics; it touches on deeply personal and psychological aspects of one's identity and self-esteem.

The psychological benefits of hair restoration are emphasized along with its importance for cosmetic purposes. Readers can make informed decisions about their preferred treatment paths by learning about a variety of approaches that are tailored to their specific needs through in-depth explanations of both surgical and non-surgical options. Non-surgical methods like medications, topical treatments, laser therapy, nutritional supplements, and lifestyle adjustments are thoroughly examined, with an emphasis on their suitability and effectiveness.

For individuals contemplating surgical options such as Follicular Unit Extraction (FUE) and Follicular Unit Transplantation (FUT), the book offers a comprehensive, step-by-step explanation of each procedure. From the initial consultation to the post-operative care, every detail is carefully covered to guarantee that readers know exactly what to expect at every turn. A thorough discussion of the factors that influence the choice of procedure, such as characteristics of the scalp and hair, costs, risks, and recovery timelines, gives readers the confidence to make these decisions.

In addition to physical preparation, preparing for hair restoration involves emotional preparation as well. The book walks readers through mental preparation, pre-operative instructions, and what to expect on surgery day, making sure they are well-prepared for a seamless recovery. Post-operative care and long-term maintenance are equally important, offering helpful guidance on how to manage pain, take care of newly transplanted hair, and maximize results with proper hair care practices and follow-up visits.

In "Hair Restoration Procedures for Beginners," frequently asked questions and misconceptions are cleared up with a dedicated FAQ section. Topics covered include procedure length and recovery times, the natural look of results, and choosing qualified surgeons. This comprehensive coverage provides clarity and comfort to individuals starting their hair restoration journey.

This book is meant to be both a reference and a comforting friend for anyone thinking about or undergoing hair restoration procedures. It combines professional analysis with compassionate advice to provide readers with the knowledge they need to make informed decisions regarding their hair health and restoration objectives.

CHAPTER ONE
HAIR RESTORATION PROCEDURES OVERVIEW
COMPREHENDING HAIR LOSS

For anyone thinking about hair restoration procedures, it is important to understand hair loss. Hair loss can be caused by a variety of factors, such as genetics, hormonal changes, medical conditions, and lifestyle choices. First and foremost, it is important to understand that hair loss can have an impact on quality of life and self-esteem for both men and women. Usually, hair loss begins gradually, thinning out and eventually progressing to balding in specific areas. There are several types of hair loss, including alopecia areata, male pattern baldness, female pattern hair loss, and telogen effluvium, each with unique traits and underlying causes.

Understanding the specific type and extent of hair loss is foundational in selecting the most appropriate restoration method.

Having this knowledge empowers individuals to make informed decisions about their hair restoration journey, ensuring they choose methods tailored to their unique needs and expectations. Consulting with a dermatologist or hair restoration specialist can help identify the root cause of hair loss. Diagnostic tools like scalp examinations, blood tests, and sometimes biopsies help determine the cause and guide treatment decisions.

THE SIGNIFICANCE OF HAIR RESTORATION

Effective hair restoration can reverse the psychological impact of hair loss, improving social interactions and professional opportunities. Hair plays a significant role in framing facial features and enhancing overall appearance, influencing how others perceive us and how we feel about ourselves. The significance of hair restoration extends beyond cosmetic concerns, impacting emotional well-being and self-confidence.

For many individuals experiencing hair loss, restoration procedures offer a renewed sense of identity and confidence.

In addition, hair restoration procedures make people feel good about them. They give them back control over how they look and improve their quality of life. People who treat hair loss early on can stop it from getting worse and look younger. People who are unaware of the life-changing benefits of hair restoration are inspired to research their options and take the first steps toward feeling confident and self-assured again.

SYNOPSIS OF SURGICAL AND NON-SURGICAL OPTIONS

Beginners who are interested in hair restoration are presented with a range of options, both surgical and non-surgical, based on their individual needs and preferences. Non-surgical techniques include topical applications or oral administration of medications such as finasteride and minoxidil, which stimulate hair follicles and stop further loss of hair; these treatments are usually administered under medical supervision. Low-level laser therapy (LLLT) is another non-surgical technique that stimulates hair follicles and improves hair growth using safe, non-invasive technology.

Follicular Unit Transplantation (FUT) and Follicular Unit Extraction (FUE) are common surgical techniques where healthy hair follicles from donor areas are transplanted to balding or thinning areas; advanced technologies like robotic hair transplantation enhance precision and outcomes, ensuring natural-looking results; and seeking more significant results, hair transplant procedures provide permanent solutions to hair loss. Beginners can make informed decisions based on factors such as desired results, budget, and medical considerations by knowing the differences between non-surgical and surgical options.

FUNDAMENTAL ANATOMY OF HAIR

A basic understanding of hair anatomy is beneficial before beginning hair restoration procedures. Hair is made up of two main parts: the hair shaft and the follicle. The hair shaft is visible above the skin's surface and is made up of keratinized cells arranged in three layers: the medulla, cortex, and cuticle. The follicle is a small tubular structure located in the skin from which hair grows. It contains the hair bulb, which nourishes and supports hair growth. Surrounding the follicle are sebaceous glands that produce sebum, a natural oil that moisturizes and protects the hair and scalp.

Basic knowledge of hair anatomy and growth principles helps beginners understand how hair restoration procedures interact with natural hair biology to achieve optimal results. Every hair follicle goes through a growth cycle, which consists of three phases: anagen (growth phase), catagen (transitional phase), and telogen (resting phase).

HAVING REASONABLE EXPECTATIONS

It's important for those thinking about hair restoration procedures to have reasonable expectations. Although the latest methods provide great improvements, it's important to realize that individual factors like hair type, degree of hair loss, and treatment method selected affect the outcome. Those who are new to hair restoration should anticipate gradual rather than dramatic changes, as hair restoration usually requires several sessions and a recovery period.

By understanding that hair restoration is a journey requiring patience and commitment to achieve desired results, beginners can approach hair restoration with confidence and informed decision-making. Consultations with hair restoration specialists offer realistic assessments based on individual circumstances, outlining expected timelines and potential outcomes.

CHAPTER TWO

OVERVIEW OF HAIR RESTORATION

HAIR LOSS CAUSES AND TYPES

Hormonal changes, such as those during pregnancy or menopause, can also trigger temporary or permanent hair loss by disrupting the hair growth cycle. Genetic predispositions, medical conditions such as alopecia areata, and certain medications or treatments are among the factors that can cause hair loss. One of the main genetic causes of hair loss is androgenetic alopecia, also known as male or female pattern baldness, where hair follicles shrink over time, leading to thinner hair and eventual loss.

Other potential causes include autoimmune diseases such as lupus, severe styling practices that harm hair follicles, nutritional deficiencies, and psychological or physical stress. Determining the underlying cause is essential to developing the best hair restoration strategy that is customized for each patient.

IMPLICATIONS OF HAIR LOSS ON THE MIND

A person's psychological health and self-esteem are greatly affected by hair loss, which frequently goes beyond physical appearance. People who are experiencing hair loss may experience social disengagement, anxiety, or depression as a result of feeling self-conscious.

Hair is closely associated with cultural norms and identity, making losing it emotionally difficult for many.

To address the psychological impact, in addition to hair restoration, individuals may require counseling and emotional support to help them adjust to the changes. Hair restoration is a highly effective way to boost one's self-esteem and quality of life, which emphasizes the significance of complete care that takes into account both the physical and emotional aspects of health.

THE ADVANTAGES OF HAIR RESTORATION

Beyond its cosmetic benefits, hair restoration improves one's self-image, giving one a sense of normalcy and confidence in one's appearance. As confidence permeates all facets of life, improved self-esteem can have a positive impact on social interactions and career opportunities.

Furthermore, hair restoration techniques have come a long way, providing long-lasting results that not only restore hair but also quality of life. Modern techniques such as follicular unit transplantation (FUT) and follicular unit extraction (FUE) ensure precise, natural hairline restoration. These procedures are safe and effective, restoring not only hair but also quality of life with minimal downtime.

OVERVIEW OF VARIOUS TREATMENT CHOICES

Hair restoration is the umbrella term for a range of individually customized treatment options.

Surgical procedures such as FUT require removing a strip of hair-bearing scalp to transplant follicular units to balding areas; FUE, on the other hand, removes individual follicular units from donor sites and implants them into recipient sites, providing a less invasive, scar-free alternative.

Low-level laser therapy (LLLT) stimulates hair follicles, enhancing growth and thickness; platelet-rich plasma (PRP) therapy uses the patient's blood components to stimulate hair follicles, promoting natural hair regrowth; and medications like minoxidil and finasteride, which promote hair growth and prevent further loss.

THE VALUE OF SPEAKING WITH AN EXPERT

Personalized assessment and treatment planning requires consultation with a hair restoration specialist. These professionals assess the degree of hair loss, determine the underlying causes, and suggest appropriate treatment options based on each patient's expectations and goals. The initial consultation guarantees a thorough understanding of the patient's needs and concerns.

Building a trusting relationship with a specialist fosters open communication, ensuring optimal treatment outcomes and satisfaction; regular follow-ups allow for adjustments and progress monitoring, ensuring long-term success in hair restoration efforts; and specialists provide detailed information on procedural options, expected outcomes, and potential risks, empowering patients to make informed decisions about their hair restoration journey.

CHAPTER THREE

NON-SURGICAL TECHNIQUES FOR HAIR RESTORATION

SYNOPSIS OF DRUGS AND TOPICAL THERAPIES

The foundational approaches to non-surgical hair restoration are represented by medications and topical treatments, which provide affordable options for individuals who are experiencing hair loss. Examples of these treatments include FDA-approved medications such as finasteride and minoxidil, which function through distinct mechanisms to promote hair growth and prevent further loss.

Minoxidil, when applied topically, increases blood flow to the hair follicles, stimulating growth and thickening existing hair; it is typically used twice daily and may take several months to show noticeable results. Finasteride, when taken orally, blocks the conversion of testosterone into dihydrotestosterone (DHT), a hormone linked to hair loss in genetically susceptible individuals. This approach is more appropriate for men and requires co.

Minoxidil is frequently used in topical treatments in combination with other ingredients such as retinoids or peptides to increase their efficacy.

These combinations can address particular aspects of hair loss, like inflammation or follicle health, offering a comprehensive approach to treatment. Users must carefully follow instructions, as application and consistency are critical to maximizing results. Although these treatments can be successful, individual responses may differ, so speaking with a healthcare provider is important to determine suitability and effectively manage expectations.

KNOWING ABOUT LASER TREATMENT

Laser therapy also referred to as low-level laser therapy (LLLT) or red light therapy, has become more and more popular as a non-surgical method for hair restoration.

Because it is painless and non-invasive, many people find laser therapy to be a convenient option. The lasers penetrate the scalp tissue, increasing cellular metabolism and improving blood circulation to the follicles, which in turn revitalizes dormant follicles and encourages the growth phase of hair, possibly resulting in thicker, fuller hair in the long run.

Laser therapy devices can vary from handheld combs to caps with therapeutic light-emitting diodes. Treatment frequency varies but usually entails regular sessions, usually multiple times a week at first, followed by maintenance sessions as needed. Users must be patient and consistent as results may take several months to manifest. Laser therapy is generally safe and appropriate for both men and women experiencing genetic hair loss, though individual outcomes may differ. Consulting a dermatologist or healthcare provider can offer personalized guidance on device selection and treatment protocols.

SUPPLEMENTAL NUTRITION FOR HEALTHY HAIR

Supplemental nutrition provides vitamins, minerals, and other nutrients that are necessary for healthy hair growth and maintenance. Biotin, a vitamin that is part of the B-complex, is well known for its ability to strengthen hair and nails.

Supplements that contain biotin, when combined with other vitamins like B12 and D, can help address deficiencies that may affect the quality and growth of hair. Additionally, minerals like iron and zinc are important for the health of the scalp overall and for the function of hair follicles.

In addition to vitamins and minerals, supplements can contain marine proteins like collagen or herbal extracts like saw palmetto, which can support hair growth and structure.

These supplements are usually taken orally and should be used as prescribed to get the best results.

Although supplements can support other hair restoration techniques, they might not be enough on their own to significantly increase hair growth in cases of advanced hair loss. It is best to speak with a healthcare professional or nutritionist to determine the appropriate supplements and dosages based on individual needs and health conditions.

MODIFICATIONS TO LIFESTYLE FOR HAIR GROWTH

Modifying one's lifestyle can have a big impact on hair growth and overall hair health. Things like stress management, getting enough sleep, and eating a balanced, nutrient-rich diet are important for supporting the function and growth cycles of hair follicles.

Reducing cortisol levels, which can cause hair loss, can help manage stress. Getting enough sleep is important for overall health because it allows the body to repair and regenerate cells, including those in the scalp and hair follicles.

Whole foods—fruits, vegetables, lean proteins, and healthy fats—offer vital nutrients, such as vitamins A, C, and E, which are critical for hair growth.

Adequate hydration is also important, as drinking enough water promotes scalp hydration and overall hair health. Limiting heat styling and chemical treatments helps protect hair strands from damage, maintaining their strength and integrity.

These lifestyle changes can be combined with other hair restoration techniques to create the best possible environment for long-term, healthy hair growth and maintenance.

COMPARING THE EFFICACY OF NON-SURGICAL OPTIONS

Knowing the efficacy and suitability of non-surgical hair restoration options is crucial to making well-informed decisions.

Medications, laser therapy, nutritional supplements, and lifestyle modifications are just a few examples of the various methods that offer specific benefits and considerations based on individual needs and preferences.

Clinically proven and widely used medications such as finasteride and minoxidil are particularly effective at addressing genetic hair loss patterns in both men and women.

In addition to nutritional supplements that address deficiencies that can affect hair health, lifestyle changes such as stress management and dietary improvements can support overall hair health and enhance the effects of other treatments.

Laser therapy offers a non-invasive alternative by stimulating hair follicles through light energy to promote growth. While results may vary, many users experience thicker, fuller hair over time with regular treatment.

Selecting the best non-surgical option frequently entails meeting with medical specialists to evaluate specific factors like the degree of hair loss, medical history, and desired course of treatment. Tailored advice guarantees that selected techniques meet expectations and maximize results for long-term hair health and restoration.

CHAPTER FOUR

TECHNIQUES FOR SURGICAL HAIR RESTORATION

OVERVIEW OF HAIR TRANSPLANTATION

When someone experiences hair loss due to male pattern baldness, injury, or other reasons, hair transplantation is a surgical procedure that can help restore hair growth in areas where it has become thin or bald.

The goal of hair transplantation is to achieve natural-looking hair growth that blends seamlessly with the existing hair. Hair follicles are transferred from a donor site to the recipient area, usually on the scalp.

The procedure starts with a consultation during which the surgeon evaluates the patient's pattern of hair loss and goes over expectations. Next, the surgeon carefully transplants hair follicles, either individually (Follicular Unit Extraction, FUE) or in a strip (Follicular Unit Transplantation, FUT), from the donor area (usually the back or sides of the scalp, where hair is genetically resistant to balding).

Knowing the fundamentals of hair transplantation helps people make educated decisions about having the procedure and getting ready for the recovery phase. Hair transplantation is usually performed under local anesthesia on an outpatient basis, with the duration varying based on the extent of baldness and the technique used. Hair transplantation requires precision and artistry to ensure the new hairline matches the natural growth pattern and density of the existing hair.

THE PROCESS OF FUE (FOLLICULAR UNIT EXTRACTION) DESCRIBED

FUE is a minimally invasive hair transplantation technique that harvests individual hair follicles directly from the donor area without the need to remove a strip of tissue. A small, circular punch device is used to extract follicular units, or individual hairs, one at a time from the scalp.

These units, which can have one to four hairs each, are then transplanted into the recipient area where the recipient wants to grow hair.

Hair follicles are carefully extracted to preserve their integrity and viability for transplantation. The procedure starts with the marking of the donor and recipient areas and is followed by local anesthesia to ensure comfort throughout. FUE offers several advantages over traditional methods like FUT, including minimal scarring, faster recovery times, and the ability to harvest hair from various parts of the body besides the scalp.

The surgeon makes tiny incisions in the recipient site, taking into account the natural angle and direction of hair growth to achieve a natural-looking result. After the procedure, gentle scalp washing and adherence to specific instructions are required to promote healing and optimize hair growth in the transplanted areas. Once extracted, the follicular units are prepared under a microscope to ensure optimal quality before implantation.

THE PROCESS OF FUT (FOLLICULAR UNIT TRANSPLANTATION) DESCRIBED

Strip harvesting, also referred to as Follicular Unit Transplantation (FUT), is a surgical procedure in which a strip of scalp tissue is removed from the donor area, usually the back of the head. The strip is then carefully dissected under a microscope into individual follicular units, each of which contains one to four hairs.

The follicular units are then carefully transplanted into tiny incisions made in the recipient area, following the recipient's natural hair growth pattern.

Local anesthetic is first applied to the scalp to ensure minimal discomfort during the procedure; this allows for the extraction of a larger number of hair follicles in the donor area, which is advantageous for patients who need a large number of grafts in a single session. Once healed, the linear scar in the donor area is usually hidden by surrounding hair.

The recipient area is prepared by making tiny incisions where the follicular units will be implanted, aiming for natural-looking hair distribution and density. The surgeon then carefully closes the incision where the donor strip was harvested with sutures, and the donor area is bandaged. The extracted follicular units are then prepared for transplantation, making sure they are handled delicately to maintain their viability. Post-operative care involves adhering to specific instructions to help heal, prevent infection, and promote successful hair growth in the newly transplanted follicles.

COMPARING VARIOUS SURGICAL METHODS

There are two main hair transplantation techniques: FUE and FUT. Each has advantages and disadvantages. FUE offers minimal scarring and quicker recovery times due to its follicle extraction approach, making it suitable for patients with smaller areas of hair loss or those who prefer shorter downtime.

Choosing the right hair transplantation technique depends on individual factors such as hair loss pattern, donor hair availability, and personal preferences.

While FUT leaves a linear scar in the donor area, improvements in surgical techniques have minimized its visibility, particularly when hair grows out around the scar. Both techniques aim to achieve natural-looking results by transplanting hair follicles in a way that mimics natural hair growth patterns and density. On the other hand, FUT is ideal for patients requiring a larger number of grafts in a single session.

Other surgical procedures, like micrografting and robotic-assisted hair transplantation, provide more options for patients looking for customized solutions for their hair restoration requirements. These procedures make use of cutting-edge technology to improve efficiency and precision during the transplantation process, which leads to more predictable results and patient satisfaction. Knowing the distinctions between these procedures also helps patients make well-informed decisions when speaking with their hair restoration surgeon.

RECUPERATION AND CARE FOLLOWING SURGERY

To maximize hair growth and achieve successful results, patients should recover after hair transplantation. Immediately following the procedure, patients should rest and avoid strenuous activities to promote healing and reduce the risk of complications. Some swelling, redness, and mild discomfort are normal and should go away in a few days.

Patients need to adhere to the surgeon's instructions regarding the prescribed medication regimen, which includes pain relievers and antibiotics, to prevent infection and effectively manage discomfort.

Other post-operative care instructions include gently washing the scalp with a mild shampoo to keep the area clean and free of debris and to avoid touching or scratching the transplanted areas to prevent dislodging the newly implanted follicles.

Patients should schedule routine follow-up appointments with their surgeon to monitor progress and address any questions or concerns that may arise during the recovery process. The transplanted hair may shed temporarily during the first few weeks after surgery before entering a resting phase. This shedding is a normal part of the hair growth cycle and should not cause concern as new hair growth usually begins within a few months.

CHAPTER FIVE

SELECTING THE BEST HAIR RESTORATION TECHNIQUE

THINGS TO THINK ABOUT BEFORE SELECTING

Several factors are important to take into account when deciding which hair restoration procedure is best for each individual. First and foremost, you need to evaluate the level of hair loss and the desired result. Different procedures address different degrees of hair loss, ranging from mild thinning to severe balding, so it's important to know where you fall on this spectrum. Next, you should think about your general health and any conditions that may affect the procedure or its results.

Finally, speaking with a qualified hair restoration specialist can help you determine whether you're a good candidate for surgery or if non-surgical options might be a better option.

Aside from lifestyle considerations like your daily schedule and personal preferences, you should also think about the long-term maintenance required for various procedures. While some methods offer permanent results, others may require ongoing treatments to maintain effectiveness. By carefully weighing these factors, you can make an informed decision that fits your expectations and goals for hair restoration. Surgical procedures may require recovery time, while non-surgical treatments may be less invasive and require shorter recovery times.

PROCESS OF CONSULTATION AND EVALUATION

A specialist will examine your scalp and hair to determine the extent of hair loss, evaluate the quality of your remaining hair, and discuss your restoration goals during your consultation. If necessary, they will also review your medical history and perform additional tests to ensure you're a suitable candidate for the procedure of your choice. The consultation and evaluation process is an important step in any hair restoration journey, offering an opportunity for detailed assessment and personalized recommendations.

Additionally, the consultation enables a thorough discussion of all available treatment options. Whether you are thinking about non-surgical treatments like laser therapy or topical medications, or surgical methods like follicular unit transplantation (FUT) or follicular unit extraction (FUE), the specialist will go over the advantages, possible risks, and expected outcomes of each option. This individualized approach guarantees that you are well informed and comfortable with the chosen treatment plan before moving forward.

You will receive a personalized treatment plan after the evaluation that is designed to meet your specific needs and preferences. This plan may contain information about what to expect during the procedure, how long recovery is expected, and how to take care of yourself afterward. By actively engaging in the consultation and evaluation process, you will be able to make an informed decision and create reasonable expectations for your hair restoration journey.

UNDERSTANDING THE FEATURES OF THE SCALP AND HAIR

To choose the best hair restoration procedure, it is essential to understand your scalp and the characteristics of your hair. Your scalp's condition, which includes skin type, thickness, and elasticity, can affect the viability and success of various treatments.

For example, people with tight skin on their scalps may find it difficult to use certain surgical techniques, while people with more lax skin may have more options.

Texture, color, and density are important factors as well. FUT and FUE procedures require sufficient donor hair availability, which is determined by hair density and donor site quality. The kind of hair loss pattern you have—male or female pattern baldness, alopecia areata, or another condition—will determine the best course of treatment.

When these factors are thoroughly evaluated in the consultation phase, the procedure that is selected will be customized to your specific scalp and hair characteristics. This individualized approach increases the possibility of natural-looking results that go well with your overall look. By working closely with your specialist and being aware of these subtleties, you can start your hair restoration journey with clarity and confidence.

BUDGETING AND COST ISSUES

When selecting a hair restoration procedure, cost plays a major role in determining the type of treatment you choose as well as how happy you are with the final result. Surgical procedures such as FUT and FUE usually have higher initial costs because of the specialized equipment, medical knowledge, and complexity of the procedure itself. Non-surgical options like topical treatments or laser therapy may be less expensive, but they may not be as effective or long-lasting.

Understanding these financial commitments upfront allows you to plan accordingly and avoid unforeseen expenses along the way. When budgeting for hair restoration, it's important to take into account both the upfront costs as well as any potential long-term expenses. Surgical procedures might need additional sessions for optimal results or ongoing maintenance to address further hair loss over time. On the other hand, non-surgical treatments might involve recurring costs for medications or follow-up appointments.

Additionally, talk to your hair restoration specialist about financing options; some clinics offer payment plans or financing programs to make costs easier to manage. When you match your budget with reasonable expectations for results and upkeep, you'll be able to make an informed decision that puts your desired outcome and your financial well-being first.

BENEFITS AND RISKS OF EVERY PROCEDURE

The potential for significant hair density restoration and long-lasting results are offered by surgical methods like FUT and FUE, but they also come with risks like scarring, potential discomfort at the donor site, and a recovery period that may require time away from work or social activities. It is important to consider the pros and cons of each option before undergoing any hair restoration procedure.

In terms of immediate risks and downtime, non-surgical treatments such as topical medications or laser therapy are more favorable for people with early-stage hair loss or those looking for less invasive solutions; however, their efficacy varies and maintenance treatment may be required.

Furthermore, take into account the psychological and emotional advantages of hair restoration. For many people, regaining hair density can enhance their self-esteem and quality of life, which has a positive effect on social interactions and general well-being. By being aware of these advantages in addition to the procedural risks, you can make an informed decision that fits your objectives and expectations.

You can choose the hair restoration method that best meets your needs by doing your homework on each procedure, talking with a qualified specialist about your concerns, and considering the pros and cons in light of your particular situation. By making an educated decision, you can be sure that you start down the path to thicker, fuller hair with reasonable expectations and a clear understanding of what each procedure entails.

CHAPTER SIX

GETTING READY FOR HAIR RESTORATION

GETTING READY EMOTIONALLY AND MENTALLY

In addition to physical preparation, preparing for hair restoration surgery also entails mental and emotional preparation. Since many patients undergoing hair restoration have experienced significant hair loss, which can negatively impact their confidence and self-esteem, it is important to address any anxieties or concerns about the procedure in advance.

This preparation often involves meeting with the hair restoration specialist to discuss realistic expectations and outcomes; being aware of the procedure's limitations and possible outcomes can help manage anxiety; and getting emotional support from friends, family, or support groups can help ease the patient's mind.

A positive mindset and preparedness for the procedure ahead can be ensured by visualizing the desired outcome and, for some, by looking at before-and-after photos of others who have undergone similar procedures to get a realistic sense of what to expect. Additionally, adopting relaxation techniques like deep breathing or meditation can help manage pre-surgery stress. In summary, mental and emotional preparation is an essential part of the hair restoration journey.

BEFORE SURGERY, PHYSICAL PREPARATION

Before having hair restoration surgery, there are a few physical preparations that must be made. Firstly, you should adhere to any instructions that may be given by the hair restoration clinic or surgeon. These instructions may include advice on which medications to avoid, dietary restrictions, or lifestyle modifications. Secondly, you should maintain overall health by eating a balanced diet and drinking plenty of water. These actions will help the body heal after the surgery.

Wearing comfortable clothing and making transportation arrangements to and from the clinic are practical considerations on the day of surgery. Certain clinics advise shampooing the hair the night before or the morning of the procedure to reduce the risk of infection and guarantee a clean surgical site. Refusing alcohol and smoking in the days preceding the procedure can also help improve the healing process. Being aware of these physical preparations and following through on them can help ensure a more comfortable surgical experience and improve recovery.

COMPREHENDING THE PROCESS TIMETABLE

From consultation to recovery, hair restoration procedures usually follow a structured timeline consisting of multiple phases. The first phase is consultation, where you meet with the hair restoration specialist to discuss your goals, evaluate your candidacy, and plan the procedure. This is an important time to set realistic expectations and learn about the specific technique that will be used, such as follicular unit extraction (FUE) or transplantation (FUT).

There is a recovery phase after surgery during which patients are advised on post-operative care, including wound care, medication management, and activity restrictions. Over the weeks and months following surgery, new hair growth gradually occurs, and patients can typically see initial results within several months to a year, with full results becoming apparent over time. Knowledge of this timeline helps patients prepare for each step of the journey toward hair restoration. The actual procedure day involves preparations such as anesthesia administration and donor hair extraction or preparation, depending on the chosen technique. The duration of the surgery can vary based on the severity of hair loss and the complexity of the procedure.

HAVING REASONABLE EXPECTATIONS FOR YOUR RECOVERY

Anyone thinking about hair restoration surgery needs to have realistic expectations about their recovery. Although the procedure is a big step toward regaining hair density and appearance, recovery takes time and patience. Following the surgeon's post-operative care instructions is essential for maximizing healing and minimizing complications. Following surgery, mild discomfort, swelling, and scabbing around the treated areas are normal.

Setting realistic recovery expectations allows people to go into the process with a positive outlook and a clear understanding of what to expect. It's important to understand that hair growth after surgery is gradual and varies from person to person. While some people may see early signs of new growth within a few months, full results may take up to a year or longer to become fully evident. Managing expectations during this period involves understanding that initial results may involve the shedding of transplanted hair before new growth cycles begin. Regular follow-up appointments with the hair restoration specialist can provide reassurance and, if necessary, adjustments to the treatment plan.

PRE-OPERATIVE GUIDELINES AND INVENTORY

Patients undergoing hair restoration surgery are provided with specific pre-operative instructions and checklists by their hair restoration clinic or surgeon. The purpose of these instructions is to make sure the procedure proceeds without a hitch and that the patient is suitably prepared, both mentally and physically. Examples of pre-operative instructions that are commonly provided include recommendations for dietary restrictions, medication adjustments, and lifestyle modifications.

To reduce bleeding and complications during surgery, patients are typically advised to refrain from taking certain medications, such as herbal supplements and blood thinners, in the days preceding the procedure. Clinics also frequently provide patients with a checklist of items that they should bring on the day of surgery, including comfortable clothing, personal identification, and any necessary paperwork or consent forms. Carefully following these instructions helps patients feel less stressed on the day of surgery and supports optimal surgical outcomes.

Preparing for hair restoration surgery involves more than just knowing and following checklists and pre-operative instructions; by doing so, patients can help ensure a smooth surgical experience and good hair restoration outcomes.

CHAPTER SEVEN

WHILE THE HAIR RESTORATION PROCESS IS UNDERWAY

A COMPREHENSIVE RUNDOWN OF SURGERY DAY

You must arrive at the clinic on the day of your hair restoration procedure relaxed and prepared. Usually, the procedure will begin with a brief consultation during which your surgeon will go over the specifics of the procedure and address any last-minute questions. Once you are ready, you will be taken to the operating room where the surgical team will take care of you and ensure that you are comfortable. The procedure will usually start with the application of local anesthesia to numb the donor and recipient areas of your scalp, ensuring that you are pain-free throughout.

The surgeon will then use either follicular unit transplantation (FUT) or follicular unit extraction (FUE) techniques to harvest donor hair follicles from a suitable area, usually the back of your scalp. FUT involves removing a strip of tissue containing hair follicles, whereas FUE extracts individual follicular units directly from the scalp, which are then painstakingly prepared under a microscope for transplantation.

To ensure natural-looking hair growth patterns, the surgeon carefully places each graft into the recipient sites, which are tiny incisions made on the balding or thinning areas of your scalp. During the procedure, you may be given breaks to stretch and relax. After all of the grafts are transplanted, the surgical team will give you instructions on how to care for yourself after the procedure and set up a follow-up appointment to check on your progress.

ANTICIPATIONS DURING ANAESTHESIA

Anesthesia is essential for your comfort and safety during a hair restoration procedure. It is usually administered locally, numbing the areas that are being treated.

The anesthesia team will answer any questions you may have and explain the process before administering the anesthesia, which is then carefully injected into the scalp to ensure you are not in pain during the surgery.

A slight tingling or pressure at the injection site may occur as the anesthesia takes effect, but this will pass quickly. The anesthesia team will keep an eye on your vital signs throughout the procedure to make sure you are stable and comfortable. They will also be alert to any signs of discomfort and will adjust the anesthesia levels as needed to keep you comfortable.

The anesthesia wears off gradually after the procedure; you may have mild discomfort or temporary numbness at the donor and recipient sites, but this usually goes away in a few hours. You can effectively manage any discomfort that may remain by adhering to post-operative care instructions, which include taking prescribed medications and avoiding strenuous activities.

THE SURGICAL TEAM'S FUNCTION

A skilled surgeon with expertise in hair transplantation leads a specialized surgical team that works together to ensure both patient safety and optimal results during a hair restoration procedure. The surgeon's responsibilities include planning the procedure, creating the hairline, and precisely performing the surgical techniques.

Trained surgical technicians support the surgeon by performing graft preparation and transplantation; under a microscope, they painstakingly dissect and prepare the donor hair follicles to ensure graft viability and quality. They also help place the grafts into the recipient sites by the surgeon's design, which helps to mimic natural hair growth.

To ensure your comfort and safety throughout the procedure, an anesthesia team is also present to administer and monitor anesthesia.

CONTROLLING UNEASE THROUGHOUT THE PROCESS

To ensure that you have a positive experience, the surgical team will numb the donor and recipient areas of your scalp with local anesthesia before beginning the procedure. This will keep you from experiencing pain during the extraction and transplantation processes.

You shouldn't feel any pain during the procedure, but you might feel a slight pulling or pressure as the surgeon works. If you do feel uncomfortable at any point, it's important to let the surgical team know so they can change the anesthesia or suggest other ways to improve your comfort, like moving around or taking breaks.

The surgical team will provide pain management instructions, including prescribed medications if necessary, to help alleviate any post-operative discomfort; adhering to these instructions diligently will promote healing and reduce discomfort as you recover. Mild discomfort or soreness at the donor and recipient sites is normal following the procedure.

MAINTAINING HYGIENE AND SAFETY IN THE OPERATING ROOM

During a hair restoration procedure, the surgical team adheres to strict protocols to create a sterile environment, which includes wearing sterile gowns, gloves, masks, and caps to minimize the risk of contamination. Maintaining safety and sterility in the operating room is critical to preventing infections and ensuring optimal outcomes.

Disposable items are used whenever possible to further reduce the risk of infection. The operating room is thoroughly cleaned and disinfected before the procedure begins. Surgical instruments and equipment are sterilized using autoclaves or other approved methods to eliminate bacteria and pathogens.

CHAPTER EIGHT

THE PHASE OF RECUPERATION FOLLOWING HAIR RESTORATION

QUICK POST-OPERATIVE TREATMENT

Following a hair restoration procedure, it is important to take immediate post-operative care to minimize discomfort and ensure optimal healing. Following surgery, you may have some swelling and discomfort around the scalp. Your healthcare provider will usually give you specific instructions on how to take care of your scalp during this phase. It is important that you carefully follow these instructions to minimize discomfort and promote healing.

Your surgeon will probably advise you to keep your head elevated to minimize swelling in the immediate postoperative period. He or she may also prescribe medications to control pain and avoid infection. It's crucial to avoid touching or disturbing the surgical sites too soon to allow the newly transplanted grafts to settle and heal properly.

Finally, you might need to wear a protective bandage or cap to shield the scalp and prevent accidental trauma.

It's common to have some initial shedding of the transplanted hair during the first few weeks; this is a normal part of the natural healing process and shouldn't be concerning.

HANDLING SORENESS AND UNEASE

A vital part of the healing process following a hair restoration procedure is managing pain and discomfort. Your healthcare provider will usually prescribe pain medications to help with any discomfort you may feel; however, it's crucial to take these medications exactly as prescribed to prevent any negative side effects.

Cold compresses applied to the treated areas can help relieve pain and reduce swelling; your surgeon may also suggest certain products or methods for taking care of your scalp to help calm the skin and aid in healing; it's important to stay out of the sun and avoid strenuous activities to minimize irritation and facilitate a speedy recovery.

You must notify your healthcare practitioner right away if you suffer any sudden or severe pain, swelling, or infection-related symptoms like fever or increased redness.

HANDLING NEWLY TRANSPLANTED HAIR AND THE SCALP

Maintaining healthy growth and long-term results from your hair restoration procedure requires taking care of your scalp and newly transplanted hair. Your surgeon will give you specific instructions on how to cleanse your scalp and when you can resume regular shampooing. In the first few days and weeks after surgery, you should wash your scalp gently to prevent disturbing the grafts.

It is important to keep the scalp clean and dry, as excessive moisture or oiliness can interfere with the healing process; your surgeon may recommend applying topical treatments or moisturizers to the scalp to promote healing and reduce irritation. Gentle, non-medicated shampoos and avoiding harsh chemicals or styling products can help maintain the scalp's delicate balance and support healing.

Regular follow-up appointments will allow your healthcare provider to monitor your progress and make any necessary adjustments to your care plan. You may notice some shedding of the transplanted hair as the healing process progresses, which is a normal part of the growth cycle. To optimize the growth and appearance of your new hair, you must follow your surgeon's instructions on post-operative care with patience.

ADJUSTMENTS TO DIET AND LIFESTYLE FOLLOWING SURGERY

Eating a balanced diet rich in vitamins, minerals, and protein can provide essential nutrients for hair follicle health and overall recovery. Your healthcare provider may recommend specific dietary guidelines to enhance hair growth and minimize the risk of complications. Following a hair restoration procedure, making lifestyle and dietary adjustments can support healing and promote optimal results.

Staying hydrated is also important during the recovery period since drinking enough water keeps your skin and scalp hydrated, which is necessary for healing. Reducing inflammation and smoking can also help you recover by improving circulation to your scalp.

Follow your surgeon's instructions for post-operative care and lifestyle modifications to support the best results from your hair restoration procedure. In addition to dietary modifications, your healthcare provider may advise limiting strenuous activities and avoiding direct sunlight or extreme temperatures.

TIMELINE AND OUTCOMES FOR HAIR GROWTH

In the weeks following surgery, you may experience some initial shedding of the transplanted hair; this is a normal part of the healing process and should not be concerning. Knowing the timeframe for hair growth and results following a hair restoration procedure can help manage expectations and track progress effectively.

The hair may appear thin or sparse at first, but it will thicken and become more dense over time. Full results from the hair restoration procedure can often be seen within six months to a year, as the transplanted hair continues to grow and mature. New hair growth usually begins to emerge within three to four months after the procedure, although individual results may vary.

Understanding the typical timeline for hair growth and results will help you better appreciate the gradual improvement in hair density and appearance following your hair restoration procedure. During the first few months of recovery, you should exercise patience and adhere to your healthcare provider's instructions for post-operative care.

CHAPTER NINE

EXTENDED MAINTENANCE AND CARE

KNOWING ABOUT HAIR GROWTH CYCLES

Understanding hair growth cycles are critical for patients undergoing hair restoration procedures. The human hair growth cycle is comprised of three phases: the anagen, catagen, and telogen phases. The anagen phase, which lasts between two and seven years, is when hair actively grows from the follicle and determines the length of hair. Healthy follicles in this phase produce better results during transplantation. The catagen phase is a transitional phase that lasts between two and three weeks, during which hair growth slows and the follicle shrinks. The final phase is the telogen phase, which is a resting period that lasts for approximately three months and is when old hair sheds to make room for new growth.

Patients benefit from knowing these cycles to manage expectations and understand that results may vary during the phases of recovery and growth.

Hair restoration procedures, such as transplantation, aim to relocate hair follicles from donor areas in the anagen phase to areas experiencing hair loss. By targeting follicles in active growth phases, surgeons maximize the success of graft survival and subsequent hair growth.

KEEPING DAMAGE TO TRANSPLANTED HAIR AT BAY

Because transplanted hair is fragile during the initial healing phase, it is important to protect it from damage to achieve the best possible results after surgery. Following surgery, patients are advised to refrain from any activities that may cause trauma to the scalp or dislodge grafts. Examples of these activities include intense exercise, direct sunlight exposure, and touching or scratching the treated area.

Patients are taught how to take care of their newly placed hair. They are told to wash their hair gently with mild shampoos that their surgeon has prescribed. They are also told not to remove grafts too soon because doing so could damage them. Finally, they are told to wear a hat that fits loosely or wear protective headwear to protect their scalp from the elements during the early stages of recovery. By taking these precautions, patients can help ensure that their hair restoration procedures are successful and that their new hair grows back strong and naturally.

SUGGESTED HAIR CARE ITEMS AND METHODS

The maintenance and improvement of results following a hair restoration procedure depend on the use of prescribed hair care products and practices; typically, surgeons prescribe particular shampoos and conditioners that are intended to support healthy hair growth and promote healing; these products are typically gentle, sulfate-free, and enriched with nutrients that nourish the scalp and follicles; regular washing with these specialized products helps keep the scalp clean without irritating or drying out the skin.

Apart from the products prescribed, patients are counseled on general hair care practices that facilitate the best possible recovery. These include steering clear of harsh brushing, chemical treatments, and excessive heat styling, as these can cause stress to recently transplanted follicles; instead, wide-toothed combs should be used for gentle combing, and air drying is recommended to reduce scalp tension. Finally, a well-balanced diet high in vitamins and minerals promotes overall hair health and facilitates the growth of both transplanted and native hair.

VISITS IN FOLLOW-UP AND PROGRESS MONITORING

The success of hair restoration procedures depends on regular follow-up visits, which are usually planned at predetermined intervals after surgery. Surgeons can evaluate graft survival, hair growth patterns, and general scalp health at these appointments, and they can also address any concerns or queries patients may have about recovery and aftercare. Patients can receive tailored advice for the best outcomes during these consultations.

Tracking hair growth density, evaluating possible side effects, and modifying treatment regimens are all part of the monitoring process. Depending on each patient's reaction to the procedure, doctors may suggest extra therapies or changes to home care regimens. These follow-up appointments not only allow for physical examinations but also provide a chance to talk about long-term maintenance strategies for maintaining healthy hair growth.

HANDLING POSSIBLE DIFFICULTIES

Patients are taught to recognize signs of complications, such as persistent swelling, redness, or discomfort beyond the expected recovery period. Although hair restoration procedures are generally safe, it's important to be aware of potential complications that may arise and how to address them promptly. Common complications include infection, excessive bleeding, and temporary shock loss, where existing hair adjacent to transplanted areas may shed due to trauma.

Good communication between patients and surgeons ensures timely intervention and resolution of issues, promoting successful outcomes and minimizing adverse effects. Managing potential complications involves diligently adhering to post-operative care instructions and promptly reporting any unusual symptoms to the surgical team. Treatment options may include antibiotics for infections, corticosteroids to reduce inflammation, or reassessment of graft placement if inadequate growth occurs.

CHAPTER TEN

TYPICAL FEARS REGARDING HAIR RESTORATION

OVERCOMING YOUR FEAR OF SURGERY

Hair restoration procedures, like follicular unit transplantation (FUT) or follicular unit extraction (FUE), are minimally invasive and performed under local anesthesia. Surgeons carefully harvest hair follicles from donor areas, usually the back or sides of the scalp, and implant them into balding or thinning areas. Advanced techniques ensure minimal discomfort and quicker recovery times. Many people considering hair restoration procedures frequently have significant anxiety about undergoing surgery. This anxiety is normal, but it can be reduced by learning about the procedure and its advantages.

To allay worries, it's critical to locate and select a reputable clinic with board-certified surgeons. Surgeons answer questions about possible results, pain, and recovery during consultations.

Utilizing state-of-the-art surgical techniques guarantees results that are natural-looking, with donor hair blending in seamlessly with existing patterns. Following surgery, patients receive comprehensive instructions for recovery and medications to help with any discomfort.

CONTROLLING RESULTS-RELATED EXPECTATIONS

To achieve realistic results, patients considering hair restoration procedures must learn to manage their expectations. Modern techniques can produce impressive results, but it's important to know what can be realistically achieved.

Surgeons evaluate each patient's unique hair loss pattern during consultations, discussing possible outcomes based on donor hair availability and recipient area characteristics. Patients can anticipate a gradual improvement over several months as transplanted hair follicles settle and begin growing naturally.

To realistically illustrate potential results, surgeons provide before-and-after photos of previous patients. Patients are advised on post-operative care, including scalp care, to optimize hair growth and minimize any temporary shedding. A key component of managing expectations understands the limitations and benefits of hair restoration, ensuring patients have realistic goals and are satisfied with their enhanced hair density and appearance. It is important to note that hair restoration does not create new hair; rather, it redistributes existing, healthy follicles to balding areas.

HANDLING OTHER AREAS OF HAIR THINNING

For those who are concerned about eyebrow thinning, procedures like eyebrow transplants use similar techniques to restore natural-looking eyebrows. Surgeons carefully place individual follicles to achieve the desired shape and density, enhancing facial symmetry and appearance. Hair restoration works primarily on the scalp, but people may also experience hair thinning in other areas, such as eyebrows or facial hair.

Patients with patchy beards or mustaches can benefit from facial hair transplants. Surgeons can use FUE or FUT techniques to harvest donor hair from appropriate areas and implant it into sparse facial regions. These procedures require accuracy and artistry to ensure natural results that complement facial features. Patients should discuss their desired results during consultations so that surgeons can customize treatment plans to meet their specific needs and aesthetic preferences. By treating other areas of thinning hair, patients can achieve complete aesthetic enhancement and increase their self-confidence.

POSSIBLE DANGERS AND ADVERSE REACTIONS

Similar to any surgical procedure, hair restoration has some risks and side effects, but these are usually low and transient. Sterile surgical environments and post-operative care help to minimize risks like infection, scalp tenderness, or mild swelling. Prescription medications and good scalp hygiene can also help to manage side effects like itching and mild discomfort that may arise during the healing process.

Understanding these risks enables patients to make informed decisions and prepares them for a smooth recovery period following hair restoration procedures. Surgeons thoroughly screen patients for medical history and scalp condition to minimize risks. Surgeons provide detailed pre-operative instructions and post-operative care guidelines to ensure optimal recovery and minimize potential side effects. Serious complications, such as excessive bleeding or noticeable scarring, are rare with skilled surgeons using advanced techniques.

MYTHS AND FACTS REGARDING HAIR RESTORATION

Anyone thinking about having hair restoration procedures needs to know the facts and myths surrounding them. Some common myths are that hair transplants are only for older people or that they look unnatural. Modern hair restoration techniques, on the other hand, result in remarkably natural results, with transplanted hair growing and blending seamlessly into existing hairlines.

The idea that hair restoration is painful and requires a lengthy recovery period is another myth. Modern anesthesia and minimally invasive techniques guarantee patient comfort throughout procedures, and most people return to their regular activities in a matter of days. Furthermore, hair restoration is appropriate for a broad spectrum of ages and genders, providing effective solutions for balding caused by trauma, genetic hair loss, and increasing the density of facial hair.

By clearing up these misconceptions, people are inspired to investigate individualized hair restoration options that are catered to their specific needs.

CHAPTER ELEVEN

COMMON QUESTIONS REGARDING HAIR RESTORATION

WHAT IS THE DURATION OF THE PROCEDURE?

Depending on the exact method used and the degree of hair loss being treated, hair restoration procedures can take several hours to complete. For example, follicular unit transplantation (FUT) or follicular unit extraction (FUE) requires the surgeon to first administer local anesthesia to ensure your comfort. Once you are numb, the surgeon carefully removes a strip of the scalp (FUE) or carefully extracts donor hair follicles (FUT) from the donor area, which is typically the back or sides of the head where hair is genetically programmed to grow forever.

The surgical team assesses and cleans the treated area before providing instructions for post-operative care. The duration of this step varies depending on the number of grafts being transplanted.

Following extraction, the surgeon meticulously prepares the recipient sites on the balding or thinning areas of the scalp, ensuring precise placement for natural-looking results. The length of the procedure can vary, but meticulous attention to detail ensures optimal results, making the time investment worthwhile for achieving natural-looking hair restoration.

WILL THE OUTCOMES SEEM REALISTIC?

When thinking about hair restoration, one of the main concerns that people have is whether the results will look natural. Newer techniques, like FUE and FUT, are made to look natural as long as the surgeon is skilled and experienced. The secret is in the careful planning of the hairline design and the placement of the hair grafts to mimic natural hair growth patterns, angles, and densities.

To create a customized treatment plan, the surgeon will first evaluate your expectations and evaluate your hair loss pattern.

During the consultation phase, the surgeon will work with you to design a hairline that best suits your features and make sure that the transplanted hair blends in seamlessly with your natural hair. Surgeons can achieve results that are nearly indistinguishable from natural hair growth by harvesting and transplanting hair follicles individually (FUE) or in natural groupings (FUT).

Following surgery, the transplanted hair sheds a little before going into a resting phase. Within a few months, new hair usually starts to grow, thicken, and get better over a year. Patients can expect their transplanted hair to continue growing naturally, improving their appearance and self-confidence, as long as they take proper care of it and go to follow-up appointments.

HOW LONG DOES RECUPERATION TAKE?

Knowing what to expect from the recovery process will help you plan your hair restoration journey. Most patients can resume light activities in a day or two, but heavy lifting and strenuous exercise should be avoided for several weeks to prevent complications. After the procedure, patients may experience mild discomfort or swelling, which usually resolves within a few days.

The natural shedding of the transplanted hair grafts occurs during the first few weeks of the procedure; new hair growth usually starts in three to four months, and noticeable improvement is observed in six to twelve months.

During this time, it is crucial to carefully adhere to your surgeon's post-operative care instructions to maximize healing and results.

While everyone's recovery time varies, most patients may get back to their normal routine in a week or two. You can encourage optimal development and the long-term success of your hair restoration treatment by keeping your scalp healthy and following recommended care instructions.

CAN I HAVE MORE THAN ONE SESSION?

Multiple hair restoration sessions may be advised for people with more advanced hair loss or for those who want denser coverage; the viability of multiple sessions will depend on several factors, such as your general health and the availability of donor hair.

The surgeon will evaluate your candidacy for additional procedures during your initial consultation based on the quality and quantity of your donor's hair, your desired results, and your response to previous treatments.

Patients who choose multiple sessions usually have additional procedures after giving themselves enough time to heal and evaluate the results of the first transplant. This staged approach permits gradual hair restoration, guaranteeing natural-looking results while optimizing the use of donor hair. It is crucial to talk with your surgeon about your long-term objectives to create a customized treatment plan that meets your expectations and guarantees the best results over time.

HOW CAN I PICK A QUALIFIED SURGEON?

To achieve safe and effective results from hair restoration, you must choose a qualified surgeon. You should look for certifications from reputable organizations, ask about the surgeon's specific training in hair transplantation techniques like FUE and FUT, and consider their experience, specialization in hair restoration procedures, and reputation within the medical community.

Examine prior patient before and after photos to evaluate the surgeon's artistic approach and the caliber of their work; read patient reviews and testimonials to evaluate patient satisfaction and overall experience; and have a comprehensive consultation with a qualified surgeon during which they will discuss your goals, evaluate your hair loss pattern, and recommend a customized treatment plan that best suits your needs.

To ensure a positive surgical experience, confirm that the surgical facility maintains appropriate accreditation and meets or exceeds safety standards. Additionally, transparency about costs, potential risks, and expected outcomes is crucial in building trust. Selecting a board-certified surgeon with extensive experience in hair restoration will give you confidence in achieving natural-looking results and improving your overall appearance.